HOLISM MOVEMENT

30 DAY WELLNESS PLAN
TO BALANCE YOUR
BODY, MIND, AND SPIRIT

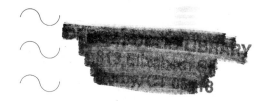

Michael P. Constantine, ND

D0840402

HOLISM

Holism Publishing
Palm Beach, Florida

Holism Movement: 30 Day Wellness Plan
to Balance your Body, Mind, and Spirit

© 2009 by Michael P. Constantine, ND
All rights reserved. No part of this book may be reproduced, stored in retrieval systems, or transmitted in any form or by any means (electronic, mechanical, or otherwise), without written permission from the publisher or author, except for brief quotations or passages used by a reviewer.

Readers should consult the services of a natural health care practitioner or other competent medical provider for specific applications to their individual health and wellness. The author's intent is to only provide information of a general nature for wellness and body, mind, spiritual balance, and along with the publisher, assume no responsibility for actions of the reader from any suggestions herein.

First Edition: December 2008

Printed and bound in the United States of America
using 30% post consumer recycled paper, soy ink,
and a green press initiative printer

ISBN 978-0-9818297-4-6

Library of Congress Control Number   2008937551

Design by Nicole Bottoms [bottoms01@comcast.net]
Author photo and logo concept: Artur Mulewski [artski@bellsouth.net]

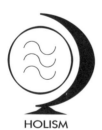

HOLISM

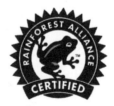

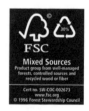

Holism Publishing
PO Box 3385
Palm Beach, FL 33480-3385
888.3HOLISM (888.346.5476)
www.HolismPublishing.com
www.HolismMovement.com

"This logo identifies paper that meets the standards of the Forest Stewardship Council. FSC is widely regarded as the best practice in forest management, ensuring the highest protections for forests and indigenous peoples."

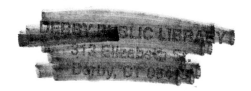

DERBY PUBLIC LIBRARY
313 Elizabeth St.
Derby, CT 06418

DEDICATION

Holism Movement is dedicated to the body of my father,
the mind of my mother,
and the spirit of my life partner.

ACKNOWLEDGMENTS

My everlasting thanks and appreciation go foremost to my mother, Johanna Constantine, for her encouragement, providence, and optimism.

To my life partner, Artur Mulewski, who awakens me to luck, light, and love.

To my father, Peter Constantine, for his fortitude, strength, and shared heritage.

To my sisters, Christina Constantine-Zecca, Marieka Constantine, and Madeleine Blake-Lockwood, who teach me responsibility, emotion, and discovery.

To my extended family of nieces and nephews for their youthful embrace.

To Maria Mulewska, who shows me there are no true language barriers in amorous expression.

To my ancestors and mentors who eloquently pave the way.

To my nine muses, Melissa Fraley-Monk, Rosanna Tirillo-Brackett, Penne Soltysik, Alison Carlile, Lori Bream-Gleason, Ivy Rose Jaqui Carpenter, Denise Perquin-Jurisch, Trudy Burgess, Ana Mulewska-Wysocka, for their creative inspiration.

To my seven sages, Richard Jaimeyfield, Rafael Padura, James McNeill, Mark Newman, Jason Andersen, Alain Glen, Eric Ronald for their brotherly connection.

To my spiritual guide Renate Moore.

To my book comrade Russell Williams.

To my book designer Nicole Bottoms.

To all my associates and clients of Immuno Laboratories who helped me garner expertise in nutritional counsel.

Conclusively, to all my patients, colleagues, friends, and family who search for health and balance through naturopathy and holism.

CONTENTS

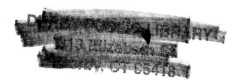

CONTENTS

CONTENTS by dimension

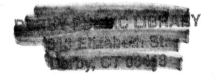

PREFACE

So too begins your Holism Movement.

This writing started with my yearning to create a book on diet and nutrition. Soon I realized that this had been done before, countless times. Despite my extensive education in nutrition through Naturopathic training and counsel of over ten thousand patients, including hundreds of medical providers themselves, the book evolved into an endeavor for broader knowledge.

Sure, I could have written about diet, weight, allergies, and immune response. It was one of my specialty areas. But the technical part sounded too easy for me, and too limited and repetitious for readers. Consequently, I embarked on expressing with word what I felt was a more authentic medicine-a wellness and healing plan that sought balance of body, mind, and spirit. Thus was born Holism Movement.

Holism is a theory recognized by Aristotle and other great minds showing that the whole is greater than the sum of its parts. Applied to medicine and health, it encourages treating the whole person, not just the parts of the body. It acknowledges the vital role a healthy mind has on nurturing a peaceful mind in health. Holism also embraces the energy of a spiritual self that lives, breathes, and has emotion.

Movement is activity and is fundamental to all life forms. When searching for a complement to the title holism, movement came naturally. It defines how life sustains, grows,

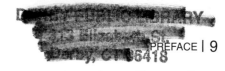
and changes. In healing, movement produces the reactions that vitalize our cells, nourish our tissues, and harmonize our organs. Our mind has movement of thoughts, whereas our spirit has movement in feelings. Ideal health strives for the equilibrium reached when all levels optimize and balance each other, and seeks a steady-state movement.

Holism Movement integrates an arrangement so that you follow one focal theme for each day. Since there are 30 chapters, the goal is to spend a typical month on the program. Many avid or excited readers will want to skip ahead, but try to follow these guidelines. It is important to awake each day with the dedicated chapter, move through the day with the lesson, and end the day with rereading the section. This method encourages you to focus on the task for good habit as you carry it into tomorrow.

Some readers may have to schedule the book program with some flexibility dependent upon their circumstances. The key point is to try to not miss a day. Discipline in health requires awareness each day.

The flow of the chapters follows a grouping by dimension. The first day focuses on a physical aspect as a premise of nature. This is body. The second day looks at a mental quality in the source of nurture. This is mind. The third day addresses a sacred element of the soul. This is spirit. Then you repeat these steps… body, mind, spirit.

Each chapter has seven virtues that represent its principles. Some virtues are basic and fundamental, whereas others are more artistic and figurative. At the end of each chapter is a summary of these virtues in what is termed definements.

You will find other patterns in this book. The cover of Holism Movement is a wave, chosen for its symbolism to nature and movement. It follows a waveform as a sine wave, the frequency also found in many of nature's movements, like electricity, sound, and the heartbeat. Waves have a continuous flow and ebb, rise and fall, just as life itself. They are continuous, and although rest, never end.

The Holism logo combines the body, mind, and spiritual elements as the earth, moon, and sun. The center of the logo assimilates three sine wave cycles to show this body, mind, spirit balance. The goal in this specific presentation is to remind the reader that life also has purpose, patterns, and natural laws to follow.

Today is the day to start a change and follow Holism Movement. Attention to health can be your direction and personal choice. Attaining health can be your reward and sustenance. As with anything to pursue in life, either you will, or you won't.

Dr. Michael Constantine
September 2008

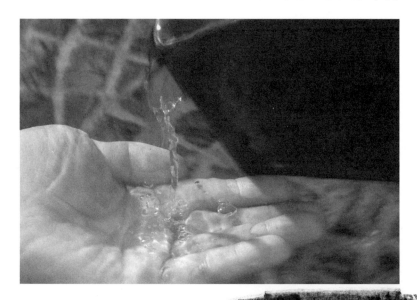

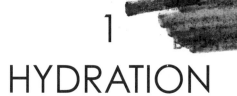

1

HYDRATION

*The holism of hydration is to fill
our own deepest ocean.*

Hydration is an essential component of the human experience, and in all forms of movable life. Water itself moves into phases of water, as liquid, vapor, and ice. The first generation in Holism Movement is for you to concern yourself with proper hydration.

The surface of our earth is comprised of over 70% water. The human body itself is made of 65% water. The primary stage of water is in its fluid environment, as H_2O, which contain two hydrogen atoms and a single oxygen atom. The fluid environment it creates is the site of most biochemical reactions in the health and being of living systems.

Your task for this day or chosen period is to hydrate yourself and your surroundings. Most health experts agree that drinking 8 cups of water/day is suitable for most adults. Considering water is also present in most foods and all other liquids we ingest, the average need may be less.

Spring water is nature's purer source of hydration. The staple drinking use of a nearby or favored spring is optimal. Most people probably hydrate best with room temperature water at the amount of 4-8 glasses of 8 ounces water/day.

Good filtered water should be fine for most cooking purposes. Noting the more usable sources of water are not highly purified, you should consider a sink, shower, and/or whole house filtration.

It is important to find your own individualized need for daily hydration. If you are drinking under four glasses a day, you tend to be less thirsty and likely dehydrated. If in this low group, concentrate on increasing your daily intake to the 4-8 glasses/day average.

Those who average 4-8 glasses a day already are likely doing the proper amount of hydration. Keep in mind on hotter days, richer food days, and more stressful days, your need will metabolically increase.

If you drink plenty, consider your true overall need. If you frequent the bathroom, or always feel thirsty, consider simple electrolyte packets to add to your occasional water intake, but not the sugary kind. Are you drinking too many non-water drinks, or eating too rich a diet?

Hydration also reaches into nature. Plants essentially need pure hydration. So do our pets and all wildlife. Again, remember how much water comprises our bodies, all life, and the earth itself. Today you should also look at others' hydration levels, including your pets, your plants, and your garden.

Think of going to your nearby body of water. This may be the ocean, sea, river, bay, lake, pool, or spa. Swimming is a wonderful way to hydrate in holism. If not able to swim, even being nearby water can do wonders for your nourishment. Lest we forget our daily bathing ritual, as baths or showers paramount here also.

DERBY PUBLIC LIBRARY
313 Elizabeth St
Derby, CT 06418

Rain is nature's hydration source, and part of the orderly recycling of water forms on earth. Standing in a light rain, or watching rainfall from the window echoes our thoughts of hydration. It can awaken our senses further into the holistic movement of hydration.

Hydration will greatly benefit your drier ailments. Here you should consider the vapor form of water- humidity, steam, and perspiration. Perspiring helps cool our bodies, and can release many impurities from our body. The use of steam showers and saunas can help activate this outward hydration. Hydration is from within outward, as well as outward in during inhalation, drinking and eating.

Our skin and protective barrier obviously require good hydration. In holism, do not neglect this outward way to hydrate our exterior. A good natural moisturizing regimen will nicely solve this aspect.

Conservation of water is a renewing presence in our human conscience. Due to the effects of global warming, climate changes, pollution and the like, one needs to conserve and value this precious resource. Consider how you may be wasteful or 'waterful' of various water uses. There are numerous eco-friendly ways to conserve this priceless gift of nature.

Move within the holism of water.

Definements:

1. Balance your water intake
2. Consider electrolyte replacement
3. Visit your nearby body of water and swim
4. Enjoy the nourishment of rain
5. Sweat, steam, or sauna
6. Moisturize
7. Conserve precious water resources

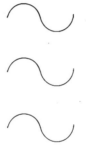

2
ORIGINS

Discovering our origins is movement
toward the meaning of life

Family is the design of our origin and the source of primary nurture. As we live, we envelop a mind of holism by first concentrating on our families. Our families are those who help to define our essence. We are only individuals unto ourselves, but among our families, we dynamically impart our being.

Different meanings will come to each of us when focusing on the wholeness of family. Yet, to understand the holism of our origins, we search our parents and ancestry. We bond with siblings and other relatives as we grow. Our friendships in life also begin to share this map with other personal origins. Once developed, our beloved is the one who likely opens up the largest door to our own self.

When you enlighten today by being mindful of your origins, who or what appears? What do family and personal origins mean for you? You should also review where any gaps occur concerning others on your given path, and those that came before you.

Think about your foundation at home. Here flows the current of your core being. This is also your starting path each day, and must be strong and nurtured. Both giving and receiving becomes essential. Even the day itself has its origins.

Direct your energy towards home today. This means spending more time at home, embracing family, or contacting a close friend. Home connects us to origins. Think today of whom you are, first to yourself. What is your desire to secure your grasp on home and family further, and therefore origins?

Even our dwelling leads Holism Movement. Structure some time to mending those weakened areas at home today. Pay attention to cluttered areas to free up space. Our head can only be as clean as our home.

In your outreach today, step outside and view the origins of nature. Sense this entire history of creation and think of how we really do all live as one. To trace nature's origins is art along with science. Nature may appear in thought, or may be drawn, visited, researched, or mapped. Whatever we do in health for holism has origins.

Maintaining your origins through journaling addresses good health. It need not be a diary, but some method to review your day-to-day living. When writing simple thoughts of your day, you create the record of knowledge to your origins. What follows is the action of your creation. You have to organize your mind, and this blends with remembrance. Keep a calendar, a health diary, or a storyline to communicate.

Remember birthdays, special anniversaries, and broader occurrences. Share your thoughts with others today.

To learn from history is to allow you to prevent repeated mistakes. Define how any areas of unease step into your life. It may also be time to acquire your family tree and learn about your ancestry. Maybe your notion is to read a book on the origins of nature, or the history of a momentous event.

Love your home and family on this day and forward. Think of those who came before you in life. Honor the source of your food and water as nature, and honor how all nourishment comes your way. Clarify your mind to know yourself and others better. Record your life and learn to map your own destiny.

Learn from history the movement of origins.

Definements:

1.   Embrace family
2.   Look to your ancestry
3.   Spend time at home
4.   Free up clutter
5.   Trace nature's origins
6.   Record your daily tempo
7.   Learn from history

3
LOVE

Love is intimate holism from the human spirit.

Spirit forms within us when we develop the capacity to love. Love is sacred and shared by higher beings. Love is the soul and depth in our human heart. Here is where all feelings emerge. Today learn the power of love as the third grace in Holism Movement.

All messages search to achieve vibrancy when they most resemble love. Whether these endowments are physical, mental, or sacro-spiritual, love awakens and opens ourselves to the magnificence of life.

Self-love is the first step on love's path to identification. Self-love becomes our identity. We sense and feel life's acceptance when our inner vision loves and heals oneself. The abundance flows over and then allows us to love others.

The first reminder in spirit is love yourself. Focus on your heart and the soulful feelings it contains. Attribute yourself in admiration, even if you have to list out your loving traits.

Love someone else today. Start with the one most intimate to your depths, as this person becomes love's truest desire, our true love. Although changeable, we only need to search for him/her once in this life.

Say, "I Love You." Write it, send it, flower it, show it, yet also feel it. For in love lies passion... the zest that keeps us youthful in living. When we show love, we receive love, and overflow love to those who miss it.

For many of us love begins in early infancy and childhood. All it takes is to spend time with children to know they incite in us the gifts of love. Our original bonds in youth then pave way to our adult and empowered understanding of love as the ultimate emotion. So too our families bestow love's freedoms.

Whereas origins help us trace our past, love sustains our future. You need to love your past and future by loving life in the present. Love is an emotion that nothing can challenge when fully expressed.

When you love your own life, you create love in others. Share your affections, and in holism, new vibrations in love will form. Love resonates with all who breathe it and creates more love.

To remember love, feel fondness for those who have deepened you. Past love should always remain love, even if the current has changed. All love up to now is still your lovesong.

Spread love today and forward to others by caring for those within reach. Others will also share this love, *ad infinitum*, as one cannot keep love contained in holism. Love travels everywhere and is endless.

Greet those you see or talk to today. Show them your love. Accept love at home with loved ones, children, and family. Even pets learn from our loving nature, and teach us in regard.

Unconditional love is to love without fault, and is only attractive when unmeasured. Universal love is to love all else.

For my love in Holism Movement

Definements:

1. Love thyself
2. Love another
3. Love your life
4. Create love
5. Remember love
6. Spread love
7. Love universally

4

INGESTION

*Ingestion of purer nourishment feeds
your Holism Movement.*

Life sustains us through proper diet and nutrition. It starts
when we dedicate each day to feeding our physical bodies
the best we know how. Ingestion also means learning what
our bodies need and truly want.

The first turn in Holism Movement is ingestion of food.
Many of us have trouble with the initial selection of food for
the day. Some will need fiber, others more protein. These are
better choices for early integration. Just as you choose purer
hydration arising the day, consider wisely what your body is
messaging today for food.

Some suggestions for ingestion earlier in the day are
fiber cereals, fruit, lean protein, protein shakes, fresh
vegetable juices, green drinks, lightly cooked vegetables,
homemade soups, and even lighter fare leftovers. Midday
meals should incorporate a denser variety of proteins and

vegetables. Later day meals should generally be lighter in portions and lower in proteins.

One key principle is food rotation. It may take up to 4 days to process your meals in entirety. You do not want to overload on any given product by way of repetition. Thus, this fourth step in Holism Movement also requests that you vary your diet over 4 day spans. Although you can repeat meals and food items within a 24-hour period, try then avoid that food for the next several days. Ideally, this means not even having the same ingredient the next few days. You will have to pay attention to food labels on packaged foods, and anything the prepared food contains.

The essence of physical ingestion is variety. By listing out your foods and all you ingest with a food log, you can assure yourself of not overdoing this spice of life. Keeping track of what goes into your body will also show its lack or excess.

Our body requires numerous and various nourishments throughout the day. Feed the day by planning ingestion of 2-4 solid, healthy meals and 2-4 nutritious snacks. Whole foods are unprocessed foods and should always be your staple meal plan with rare exception. Organic foods are also preferred when available, as these foods are grown and harvested without the use of pesticides and artificial · fertilizers, and are therefore not chemically altered foods.

Healthier protein options are toward vegetarian. This does not mean meats for all are unhealthy, but everyone should moderate to once or twice a day at most. Animal products are higher in saturated fat and denser to digestion. Good vegetarian options for protein include legumes (made up of bean and peas), nuts, nut butters, seeds, most vegetables, many grains, and even fruits. Many authorities consider fish a high quality protein. Occasionally, other animal nutrients may be necessary. Moderation is a keynote, and limitation will become rewarded. Thus the expression 'toward vegetarian' is born.

You may be surprised that the majority of your immune system revolves around your digestive system. This confirms how very crucial it is to concern your self with matters in eating. To immune yourself, you must not ingest things that are toxic to your body.

As you rotate your foods and record your eating habits, you will discover that some seemingly healthy foods do not always react well in your numerous organ systems. Note these suspect foods, as you may need to eliminate them for some time or longer in Holism Movement. Although most whole foods nourish and vitalize our immunity, some foods may not metabolize well within our own unique biochemistry.

Only a few regarded laboratories can reproducibly test for hidden food triggers. They do so by measuring your blood's serum antibodies, namely those of the IgG, IgE, and IgA immune types, respectively. Once detected, the goal is to eliminate these foods from ingestion. Often only 3-4 months avoidance will regenerate nutritional immunity.

Other toxicities to remove include heavy sweeteners, artificial foods, additives, processed foods, chemicals, tobacco, and alcohol. Our bodies become less equipped to handle environmental changes and aging when our internal indiscretions become excessive. We do not need to be purist, but selective of anything that we ingest.

Taking this first step toward vitalizing your food intake also entails sharing your food and food knowledge with others. Start by restructuring the family meal plan if you live with others. Make better choices at work or amongst friends, lending insight to them of a healthier body. Others will start to notice how lighter and more energetic you become after your smart food selections.

Learn the holism of nutrition
to benefit your lifestyle.

Definements:

1. Integrate healthy ingestion
2. Rotate food
3. Plan meals
4. Toward vegetarian
5. Immune yourself
6. Eliminate toxicities
7. Share nutrition

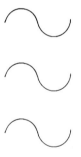

5
SERVICE

Service is movement
toward others in holism.

Here you embark on the practice of service. Service speaks the need to specialize the talents we bestow or aspire to achieve. Our deeper desires in life include the function to be a greater part of holism by serving others.

Mastery of your creative process is through development, education, and service. Before having true fulfillment in service, you have to fortify your training and master your craft. As you strengthen yourself through service, you also strengthen others.

We all develop in life by gathering our self, family, friends, community, environment, and nature's needs all into one. In turn, we communicate our lessons to strengthen life around us. To continue the fifth signal of holism through service today, you need to teach and help others master the life they lead. This mutual benefit occurs when you open up your thoughts and action for service through communication.

From this accomplishment, you can outreach in service. What are you going to do today to help others? Your home life will start this day of service. You may be preparing with family for their day's tasks, or organizing your own with others.

We all work for earnings during our life, but more importantly, for the grander rewards of service. Here is where our careers embrace the qualities of service. We all provide service somewhere, and must constantly improve on spreading its achievements. Start noticing what you can do to expand service.

Patience is required to lift our careers upward and outward. Some of us may even consider a shift in our career, or other places we perform our service. The importance here is to see the whole picture of how we are uplifting service. Heightening your potential will promote the best of service, but will require many changes along the way.

Also, keep in mind who you are serving. Do they match your belief systems and support your ultimate goals? Those you serve should uphold your integrity and share to further peace and goodwill toward others.

A final key principle in service is to enjoy what you are doing for and along with others. As you smile in service, you light up pathways for all to see. You open minds to growth and recovery.

To serve is to give via holism

Definements:

1. Specialize talents
2. Master creativity
3. Communicate life lessons
4. Outreach to others
5. Achieve career
6. Heighten potential
7. Enjoy service

6
MELODY

Melody is the sound of holism

As you read this chapter, spirit continues as you listen for this day. Quiet your mind now and hear the song around you. Is it the sound of nature or those within your own nature? Open your heart, mind, and ears today to the sixth movement that is melody.

To move is to create the melody of life. Nature's melody contains the wind, rain, voice, animals, and all life. It may start the day with a bird at dawn or a bee in motion. You may hear the rustling of the wind through the plants and trees. You may hear water or rain. The sound may be others in life starting their workday. The melody may start in your own mind song, or be heard as another's song through music.

The first sound we make in life is our first breath. Breathing begins our independence in life, yet also is our last action on Earth. Take several deep breaths now and throughout today. Feel its motion and sustenance as you listen to its melody.

Breathing is a vital part of holism health and needs attention and strengthening. Although breathing is automatic, there are ways to optimize its function. Deeper breaths create the deepest melody. A good exercise is to place or picture one hand on your abdomen and the other on your upper chest. As you breathe in as inhalation, concentrate on only your bottom hand moving outward. This is breathing from your diaphragm, and fills the majority of your lungs. As you near capacity, then your top hand should move as you slightly raise your chest. This fills the upper portions of your lungs and completes a full inspiration. You may be surprised that you have been breathing too shallow, and it may take some practice.

The full exhalation is slow, relaxed breathing outward from your lungs, and removes the last of air without straining. Let out a slight moan or hum a melody as your body opens. This is where you can start to tap into your own breathing melody.

As we wake into the day and the sounds of nature, we begin to hear and breathe our own nature. Then follows our task at hand to develop and sing our own daily song. We have a voice in speaking, laughing, loving, and singing.

Pay attention to what you say today. Have tenderness in your voice, as everyone responds better to melody. Include laughing and feel its positive effects. Reassure a loved one, and sing another's praises. Teach others your song so they too may find Holism Movement.

Melody is the sound heard throughout nature, but music is the sound heard throughout humans. Music is our communal rhythm. Play your favorite music today. Regardless of your talent in singing or instruments, sing and strum your melody. As you take action in music, you will begin to blend with universal harmony.

The pulse of your body melody requires motion. As you walk, run, jump, or dance, your feet meet the ground and create rhythm and rhyme. Some of you are quiet while others may move with more intention. The key goal is to move within your own melody.

Identify your harmony by finding a new beat. As you heal through Holism Movement, you will also hear new rhythms. Songs from the past must now blend with the voice of wholeness in today. Whether you take up a new musical artist, or genre, or develop your own musical talent, be heartfelt to stay current. The nostalgia of yesterday must progress.

You alone are a melody in life and must denote its sound and amplify to others. Writing is a melody with a flow not unlike your voice. Communication in all regards sends a melody. Continue to listen, read, and write your own unique melody.

Your melody is your own, but is never heard alone
in Holism Movement.

Definements:

1. Hear nature's song
2. Sing your own song
3. Breathe sound through air
4. Strum a tune
5. Walk in rhythm
6. Find a new beat
7. Denote your melody

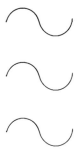

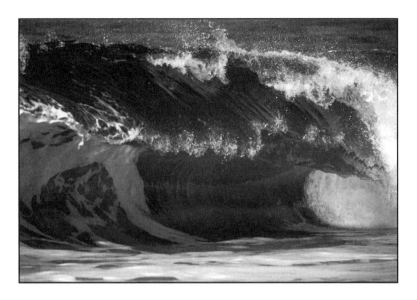

7
MOVEMENT

If holism is to embrace the whole,
and movement is integral motion,
then a new era of whole motion
is born unto Holism Movement.

Movement defines life, and all living beings have to move to live. Whether it is the simple cell in motion for food or defense, or the complex living systems found in higher animals, movement creates and sustains life.

The second generation in Holism Movement is movement itself. Let it start each day with your gentle motions to awaken. From your resting point, your body arises to meet and greet the day. Your mind begins to move in thought. Your eyes begin to move in sight. Your muscles must stretch to loosen and tighten its fibers for movement.

You will notice by watching pets and other animals how they stretch following rest and sleep. You need to do this also in early movement. Whether in bed or just thereafter, stretch your spine. Move your arms and legs. Awaken your body just as any engine must warm up. A few minutes after rest should not be challenging.

Now that your exterior is moving, turn inward to your digestive system and elimination. You have improved your hydration, and selected purer ingestion. The body has gathered its nutrients and packaged what it no longer requires.

This cycle stimulates the bowels to move, ideally early in the day and following meals. Once you stretch, walk about your initial activities, hydrate, and ingest whole foods, you likely become more regular in elimination.

This vital process of internal movement needs support through these basics. When your system is out of balance, it may need other intervention. Over time in holism, movement will begin to regulate this function.

Many of us have busy starts to the day, and for that matter, a filled weekly schedule. Yet, now is the time to reconsider your own personal movement through exercise. If enlisted earlier in the day, exercise can further awaken your entire motion. You may need to get up earlier to allow this lead. Once done, you will not skip your effort nor give way to other variables the day brings. Some of you will need a later time of day for exercise, but make it regular.

Exercise will be different for each of you. In general, you should physically stretch and relax your muscles and bones, bounce so you return your lymph and circulation, and squeeze while loosening your organs and tissues. This exercise could be an early brisk walk, aerobic activity, a lengthened stretch routine, strength training, push-ups, sit-ups, swimming, core work, bicycling, jogging, or yoga.

Follow the principle of Holism Movement. This means not pushing through the exercise robotically, but allowing the mind and heart to also open and move in fitness. Fitness requires regular health and exercise, a clean mind and body, along with an open heart.

As you continue to feel movement toward holism, walk like children. Have you noticed how children walk together in freedom and intention? You should never lose this way to carry yourself. The first challenge in life beyond early survival is learning to walk. First, we crawl in exploration of the world. We gain our strength and balance our way upright. Through effort and purpose, we begin to walk. Throughout our lives, you should strive to continue to walk like children. In this way, you will also walk with freedom and intention.

Go for a stroll in your neighborhood today and view your external life. Take a walk in nature and absorb its movement. Involving your family or another will further focus your locomotion.

Take moments to dance today. Dancing will tune you into your body rhythm and free your locked spaces. Somewhere today, spiral, bounce your body, and feel its freedom. This movement can begin alone, amongst friends, out on the town, or with a loved one.

Dancing with another helps you know them better. Be open to allowing safe others to know you. Dance with them and show them your dance. Sharing your dance is sharing your day. Draw from the melody you hear to move your body in dance. The endorphins released will create bliss as you shape your new physique.

Enjoy a hobby, as each one has a movement aspect. Your eyes move to read. Your hands move to write, draw, build, or paint. Your body moves to garden or sport. Your voice moves to talk, chat, or sing. Your mind moves to think, learn, and solve. Your heart moves to circulate and warm. Your love moves the soul.

The sacred body moves to inspire holism.

Definements:

1. Move to live
2. Stretch after rest
3. Eliminate daily
4. Exercise regularly
5. Walk like children
6. Dance your bliss
7. Enjoy a hobby

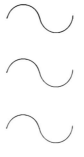

8
ORGANIZATION

The power of the mind is wise
from the holism of organization.

Intelligence in life develops mastery when knowledge learns to integrate the collective mind. Just as 'the whole is greater than the sum of its parts,' the key to a greater mind is the ability to find information as readily accessible. Organization is knowledge.

The power in the eighth blueprint of Holism Movement is to harness your mind by organizing your thoughts. Thoughts are like tiny bubbles that infuse our brain with mental pictures and maps. We compartmentalize, file, store, and retrieve our knowledge like a well-organized library.

Focus your mind today by creating a library. First, this requires you to organize tasks and goals by creating lists. Journal or write down your thoughts and tasks daily with attention to the plan of the day. This can be your day planner, calendar, notes to self, or things to remember. This becomes your 'to-do' list, as well as things you check completed when accomplished.

Memory is full of files made through association. With your list of things done and learned, be sure to organize these essential files into groups. Take time today to organize your life by filing the day.

Create a personal space to group your mail, bills, letters, and calendar. Remind yourself that to function in holism is to know where to retrieve information. Create actual files to organize your life. Knowing location is a key to memory and quick knowledge. Know where to find things.

You may first need to clear space and clean the clutter of your home, office, and personal space. An organized mind needs an organized living environment. Clean these areas in redecoration and your mind will feel refreshed. No area in your life should be unorganized. You may need a temporary treasure box to file your finer documents, papers, and objects. Other drawers, a desk, or file cabinet will provide additional storage.

The inventory of you now becomes a mental starting point. This can be any shelf you create which holds your treasures and books. You may build a bookshelf or personal library. It should include letters and photos, favorite songs and music, collections, journals and calendars. This becomes the inventory of your shelf.

You should also inventory your financial self. This is your own personal or family budget. Check your financial accounts consistently to aware yourself of all income and expenditures. Know what you have.

Continue to inventory your diet with food lists and shopping lists. Know what you eat and drink on a regular basis. Include lists for health supplements and required medications.

This knowledge of inventory allows you to know what is forthcoming and what you still need and want in life. Design a pilot board. On this board, place your dreams through images. These pictures, clippings, words, and personal items organize your life's road map. This road map becomes the golden path you wish to follow. Remember you are the pilot of your own life journey. Know your own mind.

Organization allows you to act with focused holism. You should now see the bigger picture of your accomplishments, and any stones still left to upturn. You begin to know yourself and your dreams and goals. Move forward to manifest the day. Anything accomplished today leaves less undone for tomorrow.

*Holism Movement revolves
around the umbrella of organization.*

Definements:

1. Organize your library of thoughts
2. Create lists
3. File yourself
4. Clear space
5. Take inventory of your
   self/shelf/budget/diet
6. Craft a pilot board
7. Organize action

9

VISION

Holism vision is seeing the true soul.

Sight is composed of tiny images we gather from our surroundings. What we see may be real, yet the brain fills in any gaps based on our own thoughts and life experiences. This creates a whole picture in our mind's eye.

The goal of the first complete triad in Holism Movement is to know your own self-image. To see your true self is to visit with your internal vision and external appearance, or persona. Start by looking at yourself in a mirror. Look at your self completely, not just the various parts of yourself in any judgment. What do you see?

You may at first see your physical body. This is your own unique vehicle, unlike anyone else in the universe. The form of your body has a shape, a color, a size, and a stance. This form shows your emotions of the moment, be it a smile, or a sense of wonder. The lesson is to look at your self and see the image it invokes, and then feel its sensation.

Self-feelings of your outward appearance mirror your inner self-image. Admire those traits that accent your individuality. Your goal is not necessarily to conform to those around you, or to society, but to cherish the image you are creating.

Surely, there are imperfections you now also see. What changes do you wish to make? If you see a heavy body, your goal may be to lighten your load in life. If your image is too lean, you may need to strengthen your physique and self-image. If you see blemishes, you may want to purify your nature. If you are pale, you should color your world. If you slouch, you may need to lift and walk taller among others. If you have aged, you can redefine your own youthfulness. Remember you want to change only that which does not match your own true self-image.

Once you have grasped the physical vision of your spirit and persona, focus on your mind's eye. Although your eyes relay a sense to your mind, your mind itself has vision. Many refer to this as the mind's eye, or third eye. If you close your eyes, the image that forms is the vision of the mind itself.

You may know this as a dream state, a meditative vision, a glance, or a picture. You must practice and clearly define what these images are instructing. Visual images may be helping to remember, to see the present circumstances, or to lend foresight to what may be the outcome of today. The mind's eye does not give mixed messages. It only sees the messages you have to view in holism to be at pace and peace with your own spirit.

Vision sees all, but you make the choice of what you see. You must also siphon your views of your inner and outer world. Pay attention to what you let your mind see. The world is full of woes and pain, but your outlook reflects on what you allow to enter as sight.

Change the way you view your world by also not letting in false images and harmful images. As you begin to know your true self, you see your own true goodness and beauty. Like attracts like in many regards, so do not let yourself fall victim to unwanted views. Look for the positive, the happy, the good, and the pure. Let all else filter out to be cleansed and renewed.

The intuition of the mind is the insight into becoming a visionary. Your knowledge and experiences are more than just rational thoughts. They also stem from our universal emotions. When you combine the body, mind, and spirit of your vision, you become a visionary.

This allows you to see how the past and present create the future. Your added sense is this ability to see where your path is taking you. Yet, you are not fated to follow this path if you realize an unfavorable outcome.

Envision your life by truly seeing your own soul. This is whom you are and is never changed, only discovered. What is changed is how you ultimately envision your life. You can trace where your life has been. You can see where you are today. Now you must envision where your life is going. Imagine what you want to accomplish, and move forward to let your true inner light shine throughout the universe.

Forward movement requires the inner vision
of where your spirit will soar.

Definements:

1. Look at yourself
2. Feel your self-image
3. Admire your individuality
4. Change what does not match
5. See the mind's eye
6. Siphon your views
7. Envision your life

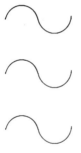

10
ENHANCEMENT

Enhancement to your physical space
announces your Holism Movement.

Our bodies strive to maintain balance between activity and rest. When the body's trend shifts toward inactivity and stress, we need to enhance our nature and strength. This first double numbered movement in holism is to correct any depletion you have.

Physically, first retrace your diet. Keep goal that food and nutrition itself enhance the majority of your vitamin and mineral needs. The broadest variety will manifest the strongest health. Review your daily diet and add this variety to your eating choices. Make it your habit each day to include different foods from the last several days.

Seek out a qualified natural health care provider. These professionals should be well educated in nature cure/care principles. Although mass information can give you many considerations in a natural health approach, your core nutrition needs to be individualized.

Some of you may already take daily or frequent vitamins, minerals, herbs, and nutrients. Make sure they are prioritized enhancements to your own unique system. Research your own responsibility to your health with proper guidance.

Nutraceuticals are the nutritional molecules that ignite our living processes. Vitamins range from water-soluble nutrients, like the vitamins B, C, and bioflavonoids, to the fat-soluble nutrients of vitamins A, D, E, and K.

Minerals contain the elements of the earth, both the metals and non-metals. Minerals to consider include calcium, magnesium, potassium, chromium, selenium, zinc, and iron.

Antioxidants serve to prevent excessive oxidation or reduction in ideal living systems. Nature and biology have prepared our body to repair its mistakes through nutrients like Co-Q10, lipoic acid, glutathione, polyphenols, carotenoids, SOD, and NADH. These are highly concentrated in certain fruits, vegetables, seeds, sprouts, and grasses.

Numerous healing plants contain beneficial extracts and cell signalers. Consider your foods and teas as significant sources of cell nutrition and repair. Otherwise, you may need to supplement for enhancement.

With the help of a provider of holism, consider the aid of a vitamin, mineral, and/or antioxidant formula to enhance your living movement. You might start with a blend, but remember you are unique in our own nutritional needs. Find the best-suited nutrients for your current health tendencies.

Essential fats provide the nourishments to the boundaries of our cells, nerves, vessels, tissues, brain, organs, and skin. The oils in our bodies lubricate and protect our very being. Humans are a unique animal ideally suited to ingestion or production of these energy storehouses.

One goal in obtaining the richest benefits of healthy oils is through our actual diet. Plants uphold a rich waxy form of oils. Nuts and seeds provide particularly useful essential fatty acids. Fish is often a beneficial choice for an animal source of omega rich oils.

If a need occurs to supplement for enhancement, consider omega 3,6,9 sources or a blend. Search for your own customized need and ratio. Nutritional lab testing may be necessary to find the best fit for your body and biochemistry.

Amino acids form the building blocks of protein. Here the nitrogen element binds with carbon, hydrogen, and oxygen atoms to form the protein components of our living puzzle.

Protein is essential for our human structure. This gives us our substance and foundation. As another energy liberator, protein forms the integrity of our skin, muscle, tissue, and organ structure. Protein predominates in our enzymatic reactions and thinking peptides. Our nerves also require the signals of many protein neurotransmitter compounds.

We tend to think a protein diet is mainly animal based, but a purer source lies again the in the plant world. Plant proteins are abundant in legumes, grains, nuts, seeds, as well as in the leafy greens and vegetable families.

Many authorities agree the basic formula for protein need, in grams, is half a person's body weight, in pounds, or slightly more if in kilograms. Even a strict vegetarian diet with smart food choices and rotation will achieve this protein need. Remember the principle of variety, as no single food serves the complex need for enhancement.

Supplements to incorporate for protein include protein shakes. Use these as a meal enhancement or replacement. Lower allergy powders are plant based, such as rice, yellow pea, soy, and hemp. Alternation of the day's choice serves in rotation and variety.

Amino acid blends can also enhance your essential need. Your body cannot make all of its necessary protein blocks, thus diet is our food for life. For repair and improvement, find your protein need and include better sources. Remember the services of holism health practitioners for advisement.

Hormones are the body's messengers to grow, divide, rest, differentiate, combine, specialize, and/or reproduce. A concluding nutrient of balance in holism bonds through our hormonal nature.

Since hormones are at the essence of our living and creation, look into the aspect of your own hormonal balance. The needs of your body change dramatically through various stages of life. In your own current stage, be it youth, adolescence, adulthood, or maturity, evaluate if your hormones are optimally receptive. Testing and counsel again might need suggestion.

A healthy body, mind, and spirit will function well on a healthy hormonal axis. Rebalancing may be necessary to alter growth, sexual, mental, and emotional responses. These may include hormone precursors, hormone glandulars, or hormone replacements. Any source for enhancement should be natural, organic, and bio-identical to the real structure in our body.

A colorful diet describes well these aforementioned nutraceuticals. Include in your diet all the colors of nature. The colorful fruits and vegetables are often the most beneficial sources of vitamins, minerals, and antioxidants. Below are some nutritional examples.

Red: tomatoes, red apples, cranberries, pomegranates, red radish, strawberries, red peppers

Orange: carrots, oranges, grapefruit, pumpkin, cantaloupe, papaya, sweet potato

Yellow: bananas, lemons, golden apples, pineapple, squash, corn, and many grains

Green: broccoli, spinach, lettuces, green onions, peas, asparagus, green beans, cucumbers, celery, avocados, artichokes, kiwi, honeydew, limes

Blue: blueberries, blue plums, blue corn, blue potato, borage, and bluish spices like rosemary, sage

Purple: grapes, figs, raisins, prunes, eggplant, purple cabbage, beets

White: onion, garlic, mushrooms, potatoes, cauliflower, parsley root, parsnip

*Holism Movement leads your body
into a rainbow of enhancement.*

Definements:

1. Retrace your diet variety
2. Seek holism health
3. Define nutraceuticals:
4. Ingest essential fats
5. Build upon amino acids
6. Balance hormones
7. Eat from the rainbow of colors

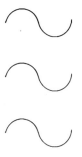

11
MOTIVATION

Grab a friend of holism and gain motivation.
Move to find others alongside your inspiration.

Today let us spend life living well,
For in a life well led rings an angel's bell.
Seize the day set forth like the turn of a season.
Accomplish all you can today within reason.

To lead in motivation starts with thoughts at hand,
So grab this friend and explore your land.
Make this day about promise and action.
You may as well leap into the day's reaction.

What is it that you will dedicate today?
Scan your registry to find the proper cards to play.
What is your goal to take into this next hour?
Which of your abilities are about to flower?

Look at your lists to see where you stand.
Follow the sunlight so you start to understand.
Loved ones nearby will help build your place.
It is you alone who creates your space.

Whom will you see come forth or meet?
You will have to go out in order to greet.
Ready yourself to venture into the world and shine.
Each step of the way, look around where you align.

The time is now to get going and speak.
Communicate by also listening to the meek.
We all have so much in life to give and teach.
Yet, you still have to learn from others in reach.

Move forward into evening, mindful of the coming week.
Each day, hour, or minute is your time to peak.
Even when the day is both too long and too short,
Look at what you achieve next to the one you court.

Today you learn motivation can be devout.
In holism, you act out every plan without any doubt.

Definements:

1. Why live today well?
2. Where will you lend a hand?
3. What is today?
4. How do you stand?
5. Whom will you meet?
6. When should you speak?
7. How long is the week?

12
ENERGY

*Energy is the spiritual force that ignites holism
into vibrational movement.*

Every particle on earth or in the universe has the chosen
ability to bind. Although energy is changeable in form, it
concentrates into selected areas where it can charge. This
creates electricity, magnetism, temperature, thought,
movement, vibration, and other energy. This is life.

From our origin lies the place in time our soul is born.
Our prenatal energy collects all it desires and deserves, but
not without error. We retain this ability to choose forever.

Your beginning as a human living cell of energy creates
this initial energy alignment. Add to this spiritual element the
energy of nature and nurture, and you create your entire self.
What is important to realize is that your energy can create,
transform, or release, but cannot be destroyed.

The buildup of energy accelerates greatly when you are
young. Yet, no matter what your given age, the building

process continues throughout life. You must find the proper positive and uplifting energy in your physical, mental, and emotional presence. This is growth.

Growth continues when we lay a solid foundation. When life chips away at this core, you must accept the need to remove any undesired or unwelcomed energy. This is change.

Accepting the balance of your nature is an indispensable principle. Learn all you can about yourself, the world, life, history, culture, nature, and how you fit into this world. You may age, but your energy can remain youthful in spirit and continue to accelerate toward life's goals. Energy is a lightening of your soul. This is enlightenment.

Our vital energies have centers in our physical body along our mental core. These centers incorporate the holism of our energy functions. Known also as the chakra systems, these various layers are energy points that serve as our main nerve stations.

The lower chakras begin as your root base and foundation. This is your grounding point, beginnings, family, and home. As you ascend in nature and grow, you develop an ability to protect, defend, create, recreate, and procreate in this second center. Subsequently, you will grow and touch the third center of strength, sense of self, instinct, motivation, and leadership. This is your youth.

In order to continue to grow and expand, your energy follows in maturation. This middle level of chakras will center on all that is love. This love needs to be unconditional towards self and others in order to evolve in compassion and guidance. When you do, you can honestly communicate to others through your voice, action, knowledge, experiences, and love. This is your power center.

Your upper chakras begin to dominate throughout the wisdom of life. When you safely and securely look deep within yourself, you see where your energy commands its flow. You then see your true inner eye that knows itself and the entire world it contains. Foresight is now accessible.

Moving upward from your senses allows you to know your religious tones and grow into your spirituality. Your energy becomes movement into its higher self in holism. This is your true wisdom.

All I can be is the best of my own energy.

Definements:

1. Your soul is born
2. Build positive energy and grow
3. Remove negative energy and change
4. Learn your wisdom and enlighten
5. Ascend the ladder of youth
6. Mature into your power center
7. Spiritualize your wisdom

13
NATUROPATHY

*Naturopathy is the healing movement
toward nature's cure-system of harmonious holism.*

Building and stimulating our vital force permeates the entire universe. Achieving this through naturopathy is about achieving natural health. Health is freedom of restriction on all planes in holism: physical, mental, emotional, and spiritual. Health is complete wellness and home to your body's natural balance.

When your body alarms you with restrictive symptoms, it is prompting change. Naturopathy can introduce you to the first of its principles, the *healing power of nature*. Also referred to as *'vis medicatrix naturae,'* this inherent healing ability of nature is vital to your primary health. It is the root foundation to the timeless healing wisdom of any culture.

Nature heals and flows with proper diet and hydration. It is established through the guidance of nature, including plants, animals, water, air, minerals, sunlight, and energy.

Naturopathy focuses on prevention, education, and self-responsibility for true health. Foremost, attention to the healing power of nature utilizes these elements.

Secondly, you must understand that to treat your ailments, you must *identify and remove the cause of any illness, or tolle causum.* At the same time, you should respect your own knowledge of your body, mind, and spirit. Take this to the aid of a naturopathic doctor or natural health care provider. Together you can identify these obstacles to cure and spark healing reactions within self.

Hering's law of cure wonderfully expresses the direction of how you heal. You heal from within outward; from above downward; from more vital to less vital areas; and from recent to more chronic ailments. So start today to recognize these facets and correct these disturbances. Remember to reclaim health through the healing power of nature.

The third principle in naturopathy involves the rule *first do no harm.* Your doctor and you should always use the least possible force and intervention in restoring and maintaining health. Avoid just suppressing your symptoms through medication. It is essential that your natural health care provider helps you to discover uniquely based healing therapies. Remind yourself a holism remedy rarely fits another in cause or treatments.

The origins of a doctor should always be as teacher *(docere),* or *doctor as teacher.* This principle means you must also be your own doctor and educate yourself in self-healing. Empower your own health. Give yourself permission to feel well, motivated, positive, and healthy. Communicate to others and professionals your unmet needs. Make sure your providers teach you, and entrust this exchange to well-being. Repeatedly, know no harm.

To *treat the whole person* is acting within Holism Movement. Nature's health and wellness, disease and imbalance, and ultimate healing are multi-factorial. Numerous reasons impart your divine healthy nature. Remember not to marginalize any lack in health. To appreciate this fifth principle of naturopathy, you treat your whole person. You do not overly focus on treatments, but spotlight your willingness to stimulate improvement. As your needs change, so will your remedies. Disregard incurability and regard restoring functionality. Continue to teach and learn about health.

A final principle in naturopathy honors prevention, as *prevention is medicine.* As you become aware of your stress patterns, imbalances, risk factors, and susceptibilities, you can instill change and balance. Intervene only when appropriate. Preventing imbalance on all levels is wise medical holism. This maintains your whole person in total health.

Nature heals by inspiration of holism healing
through naturopathy.

Definements:

1. Naturopathy is nature's universal health plan
2. Embrace the healing power of nature
3. Identify and remove the cause
4. First, do no harm
5. Seek a doctor as teacher
6. Treat your whole person
7. Prevention is your best medicine

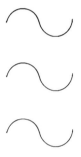

14
TIME

Time is but one dimension
for eternal Holism Movement.

Most of us see time as an unreachable dimension of life. We feel the clock tick inside as if it is the same movement for the next person. Yet, we should know that time is not absolute. According to Einstein, time travels together with space, but depends upon the movement of the observer.

We often fail to see the relativity of time. Time is reachable. We can modify our perceptions of time by the motion of a holism view.

Start by looking at the common measurement of time as day and night. This is to help you define your day and night, not to confine it to the 24 hours on hand. Experience all you can in this full day to allow exponential growth for tomorrow and onward. You can grasp time by seizing the day, *carpe diem*. Respect time as relative to your mental outlook. Revere time as the movement you can accomplish.

As Psalm 19:1-4 eloquently proclaims, "One day speaks to another/Night within night shares its knowledge." Let time be on your side. Reach it, grab it, and bend it to your will. Slow time to enjoy its moments. Speed time in discomfort to accelerate its continuance back to joy. Transcend time so you can visit your mind in all its glory.

Time is motion in your aging process. You develop yourself in phases of youth, power, and wisdom. To appreciate the infinite, and your soul as everlasting, is to understand that time within space is a continuum and yields energy. Joyful energy prevents accelerated aging. When you resonate in the holism of your movement, you master the universal law of time that rides alongside your space as spirit.

Time is a cycle. Nature's cycle shows the rhythm of the sunrise and sunset. This is your day and night. Nature displays its growth and release in the seasons. This becomes your year. Moments have their rise and fall, movement and rest. Life on earth will continue to have its ups and downs. This is the key to time, and becomes your life.

Time starts somewhere. It too has an origin. Time begins with a thought or intention. If given energy, it sparks your next phase of life. Your life can then manifest its wise choices. These choices, like time, have tendencies. Therefore, use this time of your life to create all you can be. Times change, and so will you along with it.

Time is endless and only foolishly measured. Be aware to not act within constraints of your own sense of time. Continue each day to expand your vision of time. See how nature continues its rebirth. Understand that holism sees time of the essence. Live your life as infinite, and each day as if the last.

Time is movement but only a wave in its entirety.

Definements:

1. Time is reachable and relative
2. Time is day and night
3. Time is transcended
4. Time is space continuum
5. Time is cyclic
6. Time is change
7. Time is endless

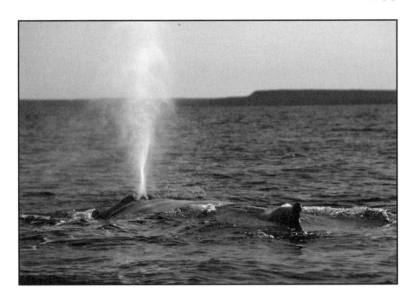

15
ANIMA

*Anima is the breath we share
in the holism of all living nature.*

We spring from nature as anima and inspire the breath of life. We exchange with all flora the vital gases that comprise our fluidity. Through this fluidity, we solidify our foundation. Our breath is nature's control of this exchange of life. We breathe in goodness and growth, and breathe out waste and exhaust.

Breathing is essential to life. Now that you have completed the first fortnight of Holism Movement, train yourself to breathe in volumes. Inhalation of pure, clean air should be full. Breath control is paramount for you to strengthen as well as relax.

View how you breathe by placing a hand over your abdomen and one on your chest. Learn to initiate breath into the abdomen. Only this lower hand should rise as you count to five. Complete the height by filling the upper lungs with an additional count of five. Now your top hand will move. Relax to exhale completely. Hold this for a second or two. Let this become your natural breath flow. Breathe in through the nose and out through the mouth for a relaxing breath, and also during any exercise.

Anima is only relaxed when you have self-control. Here lies your inner personality to rediscover. You can only identify yourself if you stop, look, listen, and relax. Your personality traits are positive, loving, helpful, and unique. Identifying the third generation of Holism Movement as anima, you lead and develop your inner personality.

As you move around your world today, notice the anima of others. Observe their expressions of energy and those you want to attract. The animations of all you touch and receive should resonate with your own personality. Whether family, friends, or lover, seek to balance your anima with others.

Enhance your anima. Communicate to others. Smile often. Even a forced smile will wipe away a frown. Laugh for good medicine. Move smoothly through life.

Challenge yourself to lift up your spirit and incite your fiery nature. Breathe and feed your fuel. Live life lively. Have charisma. Be a star.

Together, link with others in anima. Anima is not just human personality and breath. It resides in the entire animal spirit of breath on earth. What pets do you own? Which animals share part of your identity? How do you respond to their personality?

The animal kingdom is truly glorious. It is a masterpiece of creation and nature, so let this also become your focus in anima. Study and help your animal friends. They have wisdom to teach you about instinct and survival. Which animals will come into your life today?

Breathe anima with some silence today. Each yawn is a captured moment of this anima. It silences before it awakens, and carries you to change in thought and pattern. When feeling stuck, breathe through the impasse. Change is always upon you. This is what you are about to do next.

Breathe in goodness to relax your inner personality. Enhance your anima as you notice it in nature. Join with anima and then silence in observance.

Your body resides in nature. Your mind holds in nurture. Your anima follows in spirit as a third generation mover. Think of this as you lead your path today.

Nourish your spirit through movement as anima.

Definements:

1. Breathe in anima
2. Relax the anima of personality
3. Notice anima of others
4. Enhance your anima
5. Link all anima as one
6. Silence your anima
7. Follow anima in spirit

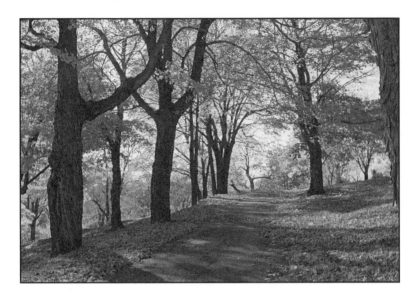

16
SURROUNDINGS

Surroundings are the holism of the world in your eyes.

Take a good look around at the beauty of your surroundings. You have explored your inner world, so now look external. Your environment is the manifestation of the world at view. To grow alongside nature and the fourth generation of holism movement, is to think of self in your surroundings. Your outward expressions literally take you outdoors in view.

The air of anima allows you to breathe in your surroundings. Admire its peace. Appreciate its balance in unison. Know your environment and its focal points, colors, smells, sounds, movements, and living energy. Take note of the weather that blankets you. Soak in the light of the universe. Color the darker times of day. Visit your environment and fully understand its power to wield.

Nature's beauty can also be your own gather. Cultivate the wonder of earth and its flora. The plant kingdom covers much of the lands of earth. It roots the soils and converts your spoils.

Plants provide food and nourishment and stem the roots of your nourishment. They cool our earth and warm our breath. Flowers color our beauty and soften our edges. Trees reach tall living heights and make sturdy our ground. You are always just a door away from the reach of nature's beauty.

The flora of the land beds our rivers, lakes and oceans. Plants meet upward into the sky and heaven. Mother earth joins father sky in harmony. The rhythm of nature is our ecosystem. It branches in movement as life itself.

Your joy in knowing your surroundings is the understanding of ecosystem. The efficiency of nature runs on balance. The environment transforms energy into reusable sources. Its currents move as earth, air, water, and fire. Your surroundings blend as your ecosystem.

You also must transform the energies of earth into reusable forms. Our higher energies now require us to prolong life by preserving earth. Going green is to conserve each day. You know earth and nature itself needs care and healing.

Recycling means reusing and reducing waste. Till the earth. Pull its weeds. Plant a tree. Utilize with efficiency. Grow tall toward heaven along with its sprouts. Care for your home on earth. Let us lighten our planet.

Your goals and ideals in life should center on making an impression, but leaving no mark. Prosper in life as you clean your earth. Walk your path without disturbing. Rely instead on modesty and fortitude to clear your way and path.

Quiet your surroundings by adapting to them. Change what needs rebirth. Feed nature that feeds you. Harm nothing along your way. Forgive, learn, and grow from any mistake you encounter. Remember to leave no trace.

Renovate your surroundings and gain energy. Remove its clutter and free up flow and space. Your home is likely the majority of your intention. When clean, home reflects your own self-care. It allows your home to fill with dreams come true. This is nature cure.

Innovate in your career. This renews your work energy. Create new progressions that have become stale. Move up the ladder you build to serve and sustain. Wealth in your surroundings accumulates when you realize wealth is not a gift or a lottery. It is a direct achievement of reform in your profession.

As you surround yourself in the day that begins, rise to the level of your outer personality. Your natural self carries a frequency observed by others. How do others see you? Are you reflecting your proper light? Make sure others understand your intentions. Lighten your spirit in tolerance to those less fit. Shape your outer environment into its most attainable features.

Draw your surroundings as movement in nature.

Definements:

1. Visit your environment
2. Beautify nature and flora
3. Blend in your ecosystem
4. Be green
5. Leave no trace
6. Renovate surroundings
7. Rise to your personality

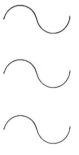

17
EDUCATION

Education is lifelong in Holism Movement.

Learning happens the moment we open our eyes in observance. Our eyes then open our minds into creative networks onto which to build and learn education of self.

Learning is a foundation of Holism Movement. We learn to hear, see, respond, and stand in infancy. As toddlers, we learn to walk, talk, say no, and train. Into youth, we school, read, write, learn arithmetic, and develop social skills.

Reading is a highlight for early knowledge and interaction. Reading should be an emphasis of all families and communities. It should provide insight and pleasure. Its value is a collection of books and drawings of lifelong education.

Reading is word, language, and custom. It is how you adjust your views of the world. Pick up your reading today. Learn to read every day, even a passage. Reading teaches you discipline, which teaches intellect.

Intellect is one of your biggest treasures. Now is the day to strengthen your mind. If in school, absorb all you can. Get a varied education in the arts and sciences. Learn to communicate with others. Make study a hobby.

Continue to train your intellect outside formal education. Research your interests and tasks. Develop your mind and find your pen in writing. Teach others your values and expertise. Expand your mind and identify yourself by your knowledge.

The highest integration of knowledge unlocks with one important key. The key to education resides in the locations of knowledge. This means knowing where to find information, whether in a book, picture, file, computer site, chart, contact, or mind itself. Your memory is vast, but most resourceful when it quickly finds its place. Learn how to reference information as education.

Continue to integrate each level of education you acquire. Store facts, not opinions, and know how to retrieve. Highlight the important principles while releasing your lesser values. Truly integrate your education and have no zero elements.

This is your point of understanding. Understand your inner world and the world around you. Uncover many modes of education. Practice your weakness while aiming for perfection. Fill in gaps of knowledge. Strive to learn more about life and culture.

At this point, try to understand others in hopes to understand your self. Admire those traits in others that you hold in esteem. Admonish those words and actions that harm. This world is full of understanding and forgiveness.

Do not bar entrance into the expansive knowledge found in understanding.

Your infinite wisdom is a collection of all your inspirations and aspirations. Thoughts and memories have movement in your mind to complete understanding of birth, life, and transition. Wisdom knows the difference of right and wrong. It expands in all directions and always stands on its own.

Focus your memory on education. What do you need to learn? Sharpen your intellect. Read with joy. Integrate these wisdoms to understand your world. Memory then finds its peace and enlightenment.

Educate yourself about Holism Movement.

Definements:

1.   Learn to observe
2.   Read for the word
3.   Treasure your intellect
4.   Integrate your search
5.   Open way to understanding
6.   Move your wisdom
7.   Remember in memory

18
LIGHT

*Brighten the path of movement with the holism
of your own light.*

Every molecule on earth has passed through a vibration of
our sun. The sun is our shining star, source of energy,
warmth, and light of day. We naturally arise with the sun and
fade when it lowers.

The sun adjusts our own body clock. It nourishes our
eyes, skin, and bones. Sunlight awakens our mind and sets
our control of emotion. This original light of the sun moves
our spirit to follow in suit.

When you develop your own inner light, you uncover
your sentient vision. This highly focused persona moves way
to enlightenment. Today you will lighten your load by
lighting your way.

Enlightenment starts with inner focus and meditation
into your inner self. It allows an understanding of who you are
and how you move through the world. Enlightenment emits

your own personal star, shining light to others on your path. Move through this day by tapping into the light that is you.

The lighted energy field you emanate is your aura. You may color this as your mood, or mental image. You fully see the light of your ways when you radiate your aura. A bright person is a soul full of light. Others will sense your uplifted light and feel its attraction. Your gathering of colored light forms a collective mind and universal soul.

Your auric field protects you from anything unwanted. Your true defense in life is staying true to yourself by shining only your own light. Color your aura to reflect who you are. Nothing false can penetrate unless we allow it by a subdued self.

Light allows you to shine. Seeing the light of day is about understanding this day in life. Then you can gleam your fullest intentions and accomplish your broadest desires.

Shine along shade. At times, you need to withdraw and step back from your impulses. Allow some shade of reflection by glistening along shade. Allow yourself to polish the shadows of others if they need reawakening. Sun and light only temporarily set as all things will pass.

Rethink the lighting in your home. What rooms in your environment need a change in light? Accent those commendable areas in your surroundings with proper lighting. Use natural forms of lighting. Light a candle to inspire your activity. Fire itself is a nightly element in light.

As you follow the day into night, begin to look under the surfaces in life at the different hues of your daily pattern. Reflected light shifts your energy field. Evening begins by your own means of lighting. This is to say the tone of the day will light your night. Visit the moonlight to experience earth's nightlight.

The spirit of lighted emotion is optimism. Your love of life and positive thinking is how you create the softest light toward eternity. Your mind of optimism yields the best outcome through faith and perseverance. Continue to look at the brighter and lighter sides of life. Keep hope as your endless light.

Since intention manifests energy in our quantum universe, hold tight to optimism and keep it close to heart. Optimism requires you truly love yourself and your purpose in life. It knows that all questions find solutions in life through light.

Life is full of adjustment and shows waveforms. The brilliance of light is that its nature of speed is the only universal constant. Everything else under the sun goes through change.

The movement of pure light will never change.

Definements:

1. Arise with sunlight
2. Enter enlightenment
3. Emanate aura
4. Shine along shade
5. Accentuate light
6. Light the night
7. Solve with optimism

19

FORTUNE

Gather the elements of holism
and finally create your fortune.

Life's wheel of fortune spins toward success. It is not flat, but spiral. The wheel has seven parts, seven fundamental elements, and moves in seven directions. Fortune can move up, down, left, right, forward, backward, or spin on itself.

Success in life is the ultimate fortune. It is not about dollars and coins, possessions, or the traits of our birth. Fortune accumulates when we steer its direction to accrue upward from the ground. Nature always fills our coffers.

Holism Movement can bring profound success. It starts with a strong foundation, furthers in abundance, requires protection, heartens by success, expands upward, values its plan, and crowns in the eventual celebration that concludes each achievement.

Strength appears as your foundation of resources. Here is the base of your fortune. You will know its strength when you find and correct its limitations. Fill the leaks of fortune by solidifying a budget. Know what you have, where you spend, and what increases worth. The importance of maintaining and following a budget is strength in structure.

In the elemental world, the metal lead is your solder. Its moveable form is molten, while it hardens to fund your resources. Use a budget to root your foundation in holism fortune. Make the strength of your fortune a base that times your pace to gather and grow.

The following glow of fortune is abundance. You have all you need and desire. You lend comfort in knowing that most abundance lies where you stand. You stand on the aluminum crust of earth, lent to build your sheen.

The law of abundance continually shows your limitless source of power. However, you cannot achieve without the blend of others. Occasionally we need the help and aid of others. Develop your financial stability with confidence in your fortune.

Your fortune requires ironclad protection. Here is where you save. You must first fund yourself to promote your cause in life. You must save for the unforeseen. Protect your finances like your home. Invest wisely. Insure things unstable. Do not cheat your savings, or borrow unvested.

Just as you armor your body, shield your fortune. Protect your valuables by always knowing their worth and whereabouts. Pray for protection, not gifts. It is what you attract that holds the magnetism of fortune.

Sharing your fortune is your point of expansion. Like copper, you conduct the electricity of fortune as a conduit that relays providence to others. You raise your level of fortune as you share your wealth and success with the world.

The charity you demonstrate is the fortune left for others. Donating the spillover of your rewards is your honor. Giving to those in need shows heart and a selfless measure of your expansive fortune. Remember to also communicate and give of yourself.

As you balance your definitions of wealth, you discover more grand treasures. They encircle your hand or hold your head with the richness of platinum. It takes communication to attract good fortune. It takes commitment to prevent these gifts from slipping through your fingers.

Honor your wealth by holding it close. Yet, open your hands, head, and heart unto the wealth of the universe. The voice of fortune expresses all you accumulate in holism.

Look inside your sterling values of fortune. Only you can truly value your personal worth and potential. Take a glance into the silver lining of your own image. The value you place on yourself yields the value the world places on you.

Polish your vision and open the gateways to holism. The reward of freedom is fortune's most valuable sight. Through thought and action, your hope for fortune becomes liberated.

Today you must achieve something to build upon prosperity. Start things you know you will finish and know will flourish. The movement of your wheel of fortune is not random. Prosperity with intention is cumulative and builds layer-by-layer.

Prosperity is precious in pure golden form. You have to mine your inner gold as you refine your talents. If you slowly build your goals to achieve triumph, you will crown the gifts of fortune upon completion.

When you reach your success, you hold apparent wealth. There are many views you will take of wealth. In the physical form starts your ability to nourish your body and home, to savor or expend. Here lies your sustenance, your health, and your luxury. In the mental sphere, wealth appears as your ultimate satiety. Your mind is without want and urgent need. Emotional fortune sails with love. You search and find your truest love. Spiritual happiness is wealth's finality. Wealth yields its movement as fire and creativity. You burn illusions to fuel your wealth.

The holism of fortune resides in this foundry of your soul's true worth.

Shine your metallic fortune
in the direction of its movement.

Definements:

1. Strengthen your foundation
2. Draw on abundance
3. Protect your worth
4. Expand in charity
5. Express your richness
6. Liberate your values
7. Crown your prosperity

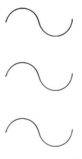

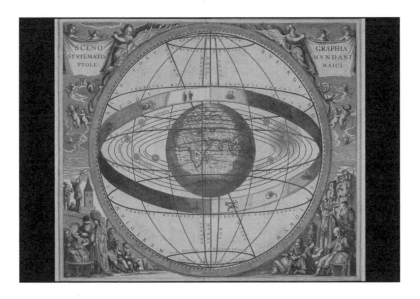

20
ASPIRATION

Holism unbound is reaching
for the pinnacle of aspiration.

Spin the rings of Saturn and remove its bars.
Then take long aim for Jupiter's stars.
Glow your light like the planet Mars.
Admire Venus for the beauty she sings.
Communicate with full span like Mercury's wings.
Touch the Moon and eclipse its fun.
Aspiration is the reach for the Sun.

Commence your discipline and planetary movement.
To exact your boundaries leads to self- improvement.
Aspiration stretches time and removes inhibition.
Now safely release your flight of personal ambition.

Aspiration continues to expand toward mind.
Prosper in life through seek and find.
Open the door to your planet of heaven.
Travel your world with these rules of seven.

Initiation begins with activity and strength.
Passion for achievement extends at arm's length.
Use dynamic energy to push further aspiration.
Wish upon a star your deepest inspiration.

Exchange your art and master design.
Revisit your love for the cleanest line.
The beauty and jewel of your dreams need frame.
Sculpt aspiration and mold your fame.

Focus on expressing your psyche opened link.
Aspiration amid heaven and earth lets you think.
Intelligent thought is your point of travel.
Commence its movement and your words unravel.

Explore your feelings and capture their glow.
Denote aspiration as emotions that flow.
Reflect in your home each aspiring goal.
Personality governs the tides to your sea of soul.

Aspiration shines in the brilliance of sky.
Your prophecy appears when you light from high.
Sing your tune of fifth generation will.
Heal with medicine from nature's fill.

Your destiny begins at your moment of birth.
Aspiration sharpens fate through holism on earth.

Definements:

1. Exact your boundaries
2. Expand your mind
3. Extend your arms
4. Exchange your art
5. Express your words
6. Explore your feelings
7. Exult your medicine

21
LUCK

Leap into your luck by entering
the movement of holism.

Open the door of holism and sweep in luck. Luck breezes into your life and captures what you hear as cadence. Luck is part mystery, part knowledge. Luck will now share with another as good luck.

This luck will charm the movement of its ride. Today you transform your life by shaping this luck into vision. Wrap luck around your house and home and blanket it in freshness.

Sing the hymns around you and hear their songs of luck. Follow the tunes that bring forth luck and lullaby. To listen to the sound of luck is to hum open this entire sense.

Here luck speaks its uhs and ohs, its oms and hmms, its woos and hoos. Open your ear to the vibratory sounds of luck. Clear the path to fullness and let your rhythm of luck flow in and out.

Luck may appear vague and not always nearby in spirit. The mysteries of fate and fortune are elusive to a smaller degree when you embrace the holism of luck. Look for signs of luck in each impasse.

Own your luck by knowing its presence. This knowledge of luck attracts its own luck. Believe in yourself and your ability to grasp luck and spring it forward.

Hold close to the lucky person in your life. You may be fortunate enough to have several, but there is always that one special someone who opens up your life to good luck. Cherish them to do the same as you bring them luck.

Celebrate this person by sharing in the luck of your relationship. Here lies your luck and benefactor. Your life truly begins when you meet this angel luck.

Any charm of luck can be your rainbow and its end. Your expression or token of luck summons this energy to your side. Rub this charm and charm your luck and spirit.

Do you not remember your lucky charm? You may have forgotten about luck. Find or create a piece of luck. Use this charm as a symbol of luck in good intention and purpose. Seek out new luck often. Luck is cyclical and passed to others in search of renewal.

Look at luck in your daily life. Luck may appear as a lucky penny, a ladybug, a surprise, or the last item of a bundle. Appreciate this message of luck, as it may fly into your life at any moment.

You have to see opportunity as luck, and turn misfortune into luck. Look into nature or circumstance for its reward of luck and serendipity. Shape luck toward vision and view the gifts in sight.

You are where you should be all the time due to luck. So wrap this luck around you and protect your soul. You will thank the movement of luck that is always there to surface.

Luck in holism is the star of your universe. Shine from the sky and light your luck. Gift your luck as a present to enrich.

Your luck is the number of your movement.

Definements:

1. Sweep in luck
2. Listen for luck
3. Own your luck
4. Hold good luck
5. Charm with luck
6. Look at luck
7. Wrap this luck

22
LIBERTY

Liberty is rooted in seven equalities of holism.

Respecting nature's laws is the first step in liberty. Life has its similarities and contrasts, order and chaos, mercy and demand, yin and yang. Flowing with nature will allow you peace of liberty.

Given truths are testaments to your second liberties. Your rules of life are rules only unto you. Yet, you share with others the best and true values as these testaments of faith.

When you stand on your own, you own your independence. You reach a third place of glory in liberty. You find your true journey of self-sufficiency.

Through fairness, you remain forever young. Actions unto others befit you as they bring magic to the gates of liberty. Fairness eases entrance into the path of your fourth liberty.

The scales of balance are the five points of liberty. Left meets right, up meets down, and the center within holds them all. The weight of your world rests squarely on your balance.

Justice is the statue that leans toward liberty. It holds the light that shines the way of fairness without bias. Justice sees no gender, race, size, color, creed, or orientation. These are the six full liberties.

Freedom from restriction is the seventh of spoken liberties. This freedom builds individuals, leaders, partners, families, communities, nations, and a democratic world. Liberty is the freedom to be true to you and travel free.

The nature of liberty allows all others
their personal choice of movement.

Definements:

1. Respect laws of nature
2. Share your testament
3. Journey in independence
4. Act with fairness
5. Uphold balance
6. Seek justice
7. Spread freedom

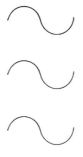

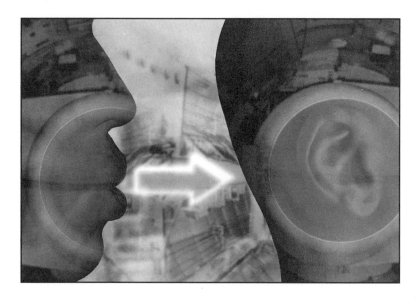

23

COMMUNICATION

Communication from a mind in holism allows
movement of the voice to follow the heart.

You spring into life as you communicate your expression. Time is anew for continued development as you communicate your body, mind, heart, and soul. Your healthy mind can freely express its deeper virtues when it acts in accord with the flow of communication.

　　Communication stems from a solid thought. Its strength in travel is through the filters of its movement. Communication must be proper and not purposeful. It should never blab, speak in vain, nor strain except in defense.

Communication is both fact and opinion. Its holism blends balance by knowing and observing the world around you. The harmonious rhythm may be a personal nature. Yet, the collective mind allows communication from the highest perspective of beliefs.

Establish mental clarity through lines of communication. Open yourself up as teacher and student. Communicate the equinox of your thoughts and knowledge.

Movement of the eyes and language of your body is demonstrative communication. Your expression outflows to others as it shows itself. Decorate your style to embrace your thought, body, and feelings. Prepare your mind with the appearance of the moment.

Your communication gathers from a place of peace in personality. It celebrates as it voices to the world. Your deeper self is enlightened as you speak your identity.

The tongue gleans communication through your deeds rather than talk. Its quicksilver motion delivers and returns movement of thought into action. Your spoken truths will register your best and higher self.

The spring of communication follows its helix through cleansing and renewal. Communicate without the need to measure your words. Shed your clutter and find limitless potential. Release your friction instead of rusting your mind.

Good communication speaks clearly of itself and intent. Better communication listens to others, asks questions, and relates. The best communication unites us all to a collective mind and the pulse of one heart.

Listen today to the secrets of nature that message your perceptions. Unblock the throat and raise your heart toward your head. Speak your fortitude through voice or pen, wish or deed, feeling or spirit of communication. Speak the language of this sixth generation.

Holism communication leaves
a trace of movement but never a mark.

Definements:

1. Expression flows through filters of communication
2. Communication seeks facts from the world's beliefs
3. Enlighten your deeper self through demonstrative communication
4. Deliver your action by communicating your thoughts
5. Shed your older self and communicate anew
6. Unite the heart of communication with a balanced mind
7. Raise your perceptions from the fortitude of communication

24
UNDERSTANDING

*Standing under holism means understanding
the movement toward peace in the world*

Emotion starts in the mind, sparks sensation in the body, and envelops the spirit of understanding. Emotion in holism is not unique to human life. Even life giving water imprints with the thoughts, feelings, and emotions that befriend its nature.

Emotion is profound at understanding the world that spins around you. You learn on the intellectual level only as you respond to the emotional energy surrounding you. Life beckons you to use your senses, feel your emotions, and ultimately know its control.

Emotion is expressive and becomes rather instinctual if repeated. The world of your emotions is vast and exceptional. Open yourself to the peace of understanding its patterns and welcoming the glory of emotional balance. You are not without your sorrow, but in holism you realize it is only a small part of this emotional balance. Gravitate toward all that is good by understanding that any pain in life is your soul's message to move away from that undesirable emotion.

Courage is all about understanding your purpose. Whether to walk, talk, learn, teach, show, or tell, courage is the ability to stand on your own two feet. You may hold hands with others, but do not lean.

Courage requires conviction of spirit to face its challenges. It requires you to look forward through only your own eyes. Understanding yourself and perceiving your honest path holds this badge of courage around your heart. You then tackle any obstacle that tries to pull you off track.

Courage is not combative and learns its strength by expressing its peace. Develop your courage to walk your talk with your own might and solemn movement. Your courage should be your offense instead of defense. Pave your way to understanding the courage maintained in holism.

Mercy lies through understanding the practice of holism in another's movement. You more clearly define your own sense of right and just through perception of others in action. This is to understand their notions, but also to understand your own.

Mercy dictates the need for leniency. Self-reflection holds strong your identity when you are strong in fortitude, yet flexible in opinion. Your views have to bend to the winds of change and allow others to pass. Permit others to find their own way in discovery with mercy on your spirit.

Equality blends the sums of life experience in under-standing our equal creation. You cannot be better than another can. You can only be the best in yourself. We all have a place, a function, and desire in this world to live, learn, and love.

Equality is the formula from which you gain the understanding that what you give you will receive. When you understand others, you attract those who understand you. This share and share alike motto is why life strives for equality to follow its order.

Forgiveness stems from this sum of mercy and equality. As humans, we err so we can learn which experiences to avoid. We do right so we can thrive within the gifts of nature. Allowing yourself to forgive the harms of life steers your path to evolve into richness.

Forgiveness may take time to understand. This is a link for your practice in the complexity of life. Forgive all others. Forgive yourself. You are not perfect, nor are any others. So, understand that true forgiveness detaches from another's realm so that you can attach to your own rhythm of holism.

Empathy lends love with detachment. We feel for those less fortunate because we identify how close our souls travel. Any of us can easily stray from the rules of life. You show your deeper respect to all by understanding the emotion of empathy.

Empathy does not take you into the drain of another. Empathy understands the greater meaning of life's messages by viewing them from afar. Understanding empathy means knowing no burden. You willingly step aside to let others change themselves toward the greater good.

Empathy is not a soft emotion but one of fervor. It allows true and deep understanding of the message in its circumstance. Empathy takes into consideration all surrounding feelings and washes them clean in the filter of understanding.

Silence is golden in understanding. Our higher selves learn much of the nature of understanding through contemplation. Sit quietly each day and at each throw of change so you further understand the world around you. Do not make haste in action, as this rarely lends an understanding.

Silence has its time, place, and season. Connect with others and the world around you, but take solitude to find your harmony. This is the true art of meditation, to understand in silence.

Silence allows you to listen to the hum of understanding. Here your emotions stay calm, your mind erases thought, and your body sits in peace. The true spirit of understanding then sets forth its silence into word.

The movement of emotion relaxes
in the way of understanding.

Definements:

1. Emotion
2. Courage
3. Mercy
4. Equality
5. Forgiveness
6. Empathy
7. Silence

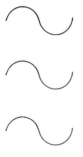

25
REPAIR

Repair is an outer movement toward inner holism

Repair requires us to be in touch with our own body and nature of our physical being. This process then allows us to pay attention to those internal and external factors that are out of alignment. Repair begins with finding any causes to dysfunction.

Examine your life and daily health activities to view what is out of sorts. What is it in life that is bothering you? These interferences are reminders of a need to repair. Start to correct how you manage your time, who you let into your realm, what you can give, and when and if you can ably achieve.

In reference to your health, focus on your weakened systems. Here is where you start to cleanse your body. Your upper body requires fresh air, water, sun, and fun. Clear away your dirty habits that impede your head, neck, and vital mind. Pamper your face upon which you view the world. Relax your upper frame, reduce tension, and move with freedom and flexibility.

The middle of your body holds your vital organs. Repair your digestion, chest, lungs, and heart. Nourish yourself with proper nutrition and remove what you know is toxic to you. Form good habits and move with joy in routine. Expand your chest and strengthen your armor of protection. Fill your lungs deeply with fresh air throughout the day. Love openly and forgive freely. Now you can develop your core energy.

Movement repairs your lower body. Exercise is your key to the foundation of repair. Walk in grace, stretch without strain, and dance with melody. Challenge your muscles with lift. Flush your toxins with cleansing fluids, fruits, and vegetables. Regenerate your vital floor by generating the energy of lovemaking.

This cleansing of health leads to the detoxification area of repair. As you remove bad habits, your routine maintains more solidity. Your daily activities now start and surround your day as eloquent renewal.

As a creature of habit and comfort, continue to highlight and pattern those activities you know restore your body, mind, and soul. The holism of repair is that it follows a path to reduced resistance. Your vital energy then protects, moves, and aligns to higher growth. Your ray to detoxify becomes assuredly a recurrence.

Repair requires removal of any weeds to progress. You must first cleanse and detoxify before you plant anew. As you repair, you can lay down new foundations and fortunes.

Growth becomes part of total repair. It does not require new creation, just a transfer of energy toward a wider potential. Replace the inertia of each day with your ability to grow from Holism Movement.

If trauma has occurred or becomes buried inside, recovery becomes the theme of repair. Change the design of injury through healing. Today may be the day to phone or visit a healthcare practitioner, therapist, counselor, or consultant. Remind them to focus on the total you, and not manage only the parts of you. Friends and family can also provide insight into recovery. This is a process that needs time, nature and patience to reach its rainbow's end.

External recovery is picking up the pieces that fall from structure. Here you renew relationships, explore newer ground, seize opportunity, and repair your surroundings. What light from your life have you forgotten? Take care of the environment. Fix your home, tend your land, and alter your path to a brighter future. All things that move, at some point, need repair.

Maintain your health and well-being with prevention. Along the path of life, turn your weaknesses into regeneration. Tune up these moving parts to prolong endurance. Your key points in prevention are to hydrate, nourish, lubricate, supplement, strengthen, move, and repair.

Preventive maintenance does not lose sight of the workings of the body or environment. Your need to tend to self will reach out, in example or deed, to the world around you. Intercepting problems before they occur cools the need of repair. Energy once again redirects to holism.

Step outside to lend a hand to others in repair. Remember children, elders, pets, family, friends, neighbors, and colleagues. Become a healer and mechanic, teacher and designer, friend and guide. Healing yourself occurs alongside the healing of others.

Further your cause to community, other cultures, and the earth itself. Conserve precious resources and you gain plenty. Preserve your body, mind, and spirit through repair of earth, human conscience, and our collective soul.

Your Holism Movement pauses
to allow renewal and repair.

Definements:

1.   Redirect interference
2.   Cleanse your health
3.   Detoxify your daily routine
4.   Grow with each day
5.   Explore recovery
6.   Maintain by prevention
7.   Heal the world

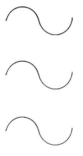

26
ENTERTAINMENT

Entertainment is the journey of the mind
to recognize happiness in holism

Days of enjoyment have arrived. Entertainment will now fill your mind with optimism and joy. Go out today and have some fun.

Enjoyment is laughter. This heartfelt emotion leaps from your mouth as one of the earliest expressions of the mind. Believe in your voyage of joy and show it through laughter. Laughter is great medicine and a sparkling light in your life.

Laughter is enjoyment. It uplifts the moods of those open to its sound. Laughter spreads easily to others. Laugh at yourself and laugh with the world. Crack a joke with comfort. Make a funny face. If you need, quiet your laughter into a smile. Carry yourself as the lightest of air in a spoken mood of enjoyment.

Level this fun and play a game. Take a lead to a softer space and claim this time in movement. Move your think tank and shake your hands. Roll your dice and spread your luck. Compete to win with a clever mind. Master your game and show others the same.

Games provide thought and pomp. They balance your learning with the sparkle of excitement. Games are a smart place to enjoy friendship and interaction. They fill your spirit with hope and a safe challenge.

Venture forth this day in a hobby. Read, write, play, laugh, view, talk, or craft an adventure. Explore your mind as you exercise each hobby. Act this endeavor with fitting drama. Experience the wonder of the moment as you create. You need to be nowhere else.

The satisfaction of your hobby builds your holism block by block. You will keep some hobbies and tumble others. Start your collection of things you enjoy. Continue to grow them in interest. Hobby yields adventure in your quest for entertainment.

The agile mind needs sport to gain in flexibility. Any sport uses movement to cross its goal. Sport for many people is a primary source of entertainment. It allows one to tumble along earth in healthy competition. Sport teaches us how we need others in teamwork.

Instead of sitting on a horse, learn to ride it. Throw a ball if not to catch it. Aim for a target to take your mark. Develop your speed and agility to spar with others and avoid all fight.

The sport of a king or queen is entertainment at your best. Pass any limits of age or time. The winners of sport always look to win again.

Entertainment is also the art that gathers crowds. Field a concert in the glory of music. Visit a gallery in the inspiration of vision. Watch a play in the company of cinema.

Dance alone, with another, or as a group in the celebration of song and nature.

Wine and dine in the gourmet of life. Food is a natural art and source of entertainment. Countless discussions or celebrations garner around dining. Food is sustenance but truly satisfying in taste and valued company.

The art of entertainment frees the mind and extends its boundaries. It connects with nature and primordial life. Entertainment maintains a feeling of youth. It relaxes the day and accompanies the night.

The height or dusk of entertainment lies in lovemaking. Affection begins in our human contact. Be it a pat on the back, a gentle touch, the embrace of a hug, or the promise of a kiss, love expresses sensation. It reaches the depths of our gifts in pure pleasure.

Lovemaking is a powerful vigor in our search of self. It teaches us to love others as we love ourselves, and to love our self as we love others. The pinnacle of lovemaking extends entertainment in its creation of energy, and procreation of new life in a new era.

As you continue your journey in enjoyment, soak in entertainment. Further your creation into recreation. Life balances its worth and success with a smile of gratification.

Join in entertainment at all its stages. Enjoyment in life sees the wonder of an infant. Games of mind play best like a child. Hobby through adventure streams the fantasies from youth. Sport of winning captures the sky for men. Art of a muse births the nature in women. Lovemaking in its maturity shapes the true adult and new generation. Recreation in its prime is entertainment for the elder.

The holism of entertainment sums
all of the above into movement.

Definements:

1. Enjoyment is laughter
2. Games safely challenge
3. Hobby yields adventure
4. Sport wins goal
5. Art gathers inspiration
6. Lovemaking begins a generation
7. Recreation delights in creation

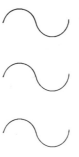

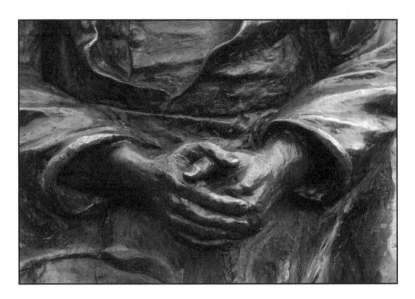

27
CONSECRATION

Consecration is the blessing on our face, in our mind, and from our heart as we follow Holism Movement.

Begin each day with a prayer to understand. Hold sacred the world's great religions, as all hold in holism the path to evolve our body, mind, and spirit. The movement you lead is as individual as you are at the center of your own universe. Holism Movement combines all religions and prays in consecration together. Here is the holism that is our shared universe and spans the seventh generation.

Knowledge of spirit is one of the oldest existing religions as Hinduism. Its traditions differentiate the individual self from the eternal self and ultimately the supreme self. As you explore the varieties of world religions, take from this path of bliss the ability to know you are spirit.

Belief in a supreme God and knowledge of self through holy law is the wisdom in Judaism. Here is where life teaches us discipline and the importance of a united family. Take from this path of dedication the ability to believe.

Life as a path to enlightenment is the goal in Buddhism. Its practice of meditation silences all chaos to explore life's questions. Take from this path of peace the ability to answer.

Traditional Chinese religions combine Buddhism with the mind of Confucianism and character of Taoism. This is where you become the scholar of life energy and venerate nature and its ancestors. Take from this path of fulfillment the ability to honor.

The existing world's most followed religion is Christianity. The teachings and healings of Jesus Christ show us forgiveness of sins as children of God. Take from this path of holiness the ability to bless.

Truth in life is the search in Islam. Its pillars instruct one in submission to God, and the daily practices of His instruction. Take from this path of responsibility the ability to give.

Combine the divine principles of our world's great religions by understanding the faith shared by all. Holism Movement is not an old religion phased out by a dying culture. Nor is holism a new philosophy that grasps at the unseen. Holism Movement is consecration that holds all holy beliefs and sanctifies them together as one. Take from this path of holism the ability to dedicate a movement.

End each day with an understanding of prayer.

The constant expansion of Holism Movement yields
new spaces to be filled by those with consecration.

Definements:

1. Know your spirit
2. Believe with discipline
3. Answer in peace
4. Fill from nature
5. Bless through holiness
6. Search for truth
7. Combine into holism

28
ALLURE

*Allure finds the beauty in holism and
crests its movement.*

The seven levels of beauty hold together and emanate our allure. Our ability to shine in attractiveness directs movement in our lives. We entice goodness so we can display greatness.

The first level of allure upholds your body's request to eliminate. The basal layer functions to release all unneeded aspects. Here is where you release waste, remove clutter, and recycle the rest. Regard this principle of elimination by cleansing your body and cleaning your surroundings. Then you become slender in your movement.

The second level of allure announces your desire to create. The sexual layer honors the source of all life and shows your intimacy. Combined with sensuality, the calm of your beauty can develop. Then you become graceful in your movement.

The third level of allure envelops your center to mediate. The navel layer supports your posture and defines your stance. Strengthen this core and maintain your balance. Then you become elegant in your movement.

The fourth level of allure concerns your approach to elevate. The pectoral layer describes your chest, heart, and bosom. The beauty surrounding here will shape your body and expand your nurture. Open your self in love and your love opens out to all. Then you become lovely in your movement.

The fifth level of allure converses your time to annunciate. The oral layer of your mouth, neck, and arms speak volumes of who you are to the world. Your presence is expressive as you move away from solitude while you talk and laugh. Then you become beautiful instead of cute in your movement.

The sixth level of allure opens your doors to concentrate. The tonal layer of your upper range vibrates your outer mind while it opens your ears. This most visible level of beauty is your face. Listen only to your own definition. Then you become gorgeous in your movement.

The seventh level of allure crowns your wave to illuminate. The visual layer is all that you see, combined with all you remember. Your higher mind will focus on what it chooses to see farther. Look not to beauty as only skin deep, but to beauty in holism as soul deep. Then you become exquisite in your movement.

Holism is beauty in its entire lure.
Beauty in movement is body of allure.

Definements:

1. Eliminate to slender
2. Create in grace
3. Mediate from elegance
4. Elevate before love
5. Annunciate as beautiful
6. Concentrate for gorgeous
7. Illuminate until exquisite

29
REST

*Clarify the mind by way of rest
to resurface your Holism Movement*

Potential of the mind lends brilliance into its next kinetic movement. Mental balance requires rest so it can nurture and store vital energy unto a new form. Mind potential achieves its direction as it matures thought into action. Where this movement will lead relies on the power of rest before it springs forth.

Build your life's potential through rest and recline. Here you can concentrate your energies in places of gather. Momentum then leaps with force and dynamism. The world now leans on a mind that can rest in peace.

Diffusion is the travel this rest takes in scatter. It grabs solitude simply to charge into matter. The strength to move through these forms of motion allows the mind to bend with flexibility and notion.

Ease your go by following your orbit. Give and take allows you to push and pull your movement. Release your mind with the outpour of effusion. Ultimately, you rest and decipher any confusion.

Simplify your life by beginning with a smile. Then look deep within the home that you find. Again, you rest with comfort of mind. Simplify this day and you will rest all the while.

Ease your stress or strain by letting go. Simplify your patterns of rise and fall. Waves in holism ebb away from exile. Go with the flow and rest in style.

Relaxation follows your action like a gift. You sit back and stretch to open it and lift. The value of rest includes relaxation from ties that bind. In holism, movement joins spirit, with body and mind.

Even the day itself needs its night. Enjoy your rest, as you soon will soar. Calm your waters to sift your sand. As your mind settles, you see the drift of the land.

The science of quiet yields the formula for silence. Your voice at rest is your song to listen. Make no sound to feel your feet. Then sequence forward with the swing of cadence.

Silence pairs with the rest of your presence. Here defines your personality in the midst of its movement. Who you become is new and reborn. Salience is what you project with cleaner essence.

The duration of rest begins as you lay your body down. Enter into sleep with your messages to keep. The benefits you reap cultivate through rest in the deep. Remind yourself that over one third of life takes part in sleep.

Your day's rest begins at your insistence. Start toward sleep as twilight begins to seep. Revisit the day's heap without a peep. Let the mind inform you of its need and time for sleep.

The outcome of rest is refreshment to awaken. A new day begins with the stronghold you have taken. You may lull into rest but be sure to excite the horizon. Greet each beginning day with determination from your path of dreams.

The journey of the dawn of holism follows the night of movement at rest. This inertia gains energy to take shape and depart. The mind from contraction now expands what yesterday had undertaken. Rest has allowed the tomorrow to reawaken.

Rest now your endeavor of Holism Movement
and pronounce your own words of wisdom.

Definements:

1. Potential becomes kinetic
2. Solitude starts diffusion
3. Patterns must simplify
4. Relaxation follows action
5. Pair with silence
6. Sleep filters outcome
7. Awaken anew

30
ECHO

Holism Movement completes its cycle
as an echo wave on the round.

So too ends your Holism Movement.

This journey does not truly end, but only changes direction and begins again. Just as an echo resounds into open spaces, the wave of *hydration* repeats its *origins*.

As you finish this final chapter, seek to repeat these steps by moving forward to a new beginning in *love*. Start again with chapter one and review a chapter each day. You might instead consider a chapter a week for further refinement.

Continue to heal with purer *ingestion* of food for your body, cleaner thoughts in your mind, and lighter essence of your spirit. As you concentrate on health, you realize it requires a dedicated *service* to holism and movement.

Rehearse your soulful *melody* to develop mastery in rhythm. Holism allows you to expand your own pattern in *movement*. Then you walk tall among men and women.

Persist in *organization* of care for your body. Rehearse your lists to train your mind. Open your eyes to the expansion and flight of your new *vision*. Practice of any task leads you closer to perfection.

When you find gaps in your path, learn ways to fill them. Use *enhancements* to satisfy your needs while you work toward holism. Improve your search to healing by radiating with *motivation*. This pronouncement of *energy* yields integral movement with amplitude.

Monthly consult through *naturopathy* fits well into the holism paradigm. If not accessible, at least treat yourself to a qualified provider of natural health care that helps revise the whole you, not just manage your ailments. The more you embrace quality health, the further you befriend *time* so that you age in grace.

As you begin to habituate the themes of Holism Movement, others will revisit you. Recognize the child, friend, or pet that asks for attention. Admire all living things as we share in nature's *anima*. Look around your home, yard, and current *surroundings* and revisit the flora and fauna of nature.

Return to your books, journal, notes, or even school as you complement your *education*. Remind yourself there is no end to learning. This book will lead to another, and then another book. Echo of knowledge responds in the brilliant *light* of wisdom.

The *fortune* in good health is that it revolves around your body, mind, and spirit. You overflow with *aspiration* when you help others. We then all hold hands together and achieve holism.

The movement of *luck* also revolves around you when aligned to your higher self. Your wish will grant abundance when you harvest your purpose. Your purpose will award *liberty* when you redirect limitation.

Remember the steps of these passages as fond moments that reshape your life. Share with others through *communication* the benefit of your find. Welcome in reception the *understanding* that as you heal in holism, you become a healer.

Remember, as well, how you felt a month ago. What has been a positive change in your life, and what is still in need of *repair*? Likely, there is room for more improvement, so why not return to this movement as a symbol of *entertainment*.

Reflect on the virtues you have read and followed. The goodness you have learned translates into wellness and progress. The *consecration* on your face emanates a most attractive *allure*.

Consider a brief *rest* if you need to regenerate your mission. Each day you vow to renew your body, restore your mind, and revive your spirit.

Echo your Holism Movement into higher ground,
with higher truth, for higher sanctity.

Final Definements:

1. Repeat
2. Rehearse
3. Revise
4. Revisit
5. Revolve
6. Remember
7. Reflect

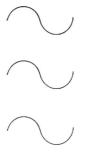

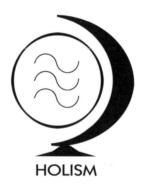

HOLISM

www.HolismMovement.com

QUICK ORDER FORM

Fax orders:	561-533-6725
Telephone orders:	Call **888-3HOLISM**
	Toll-free (888-346-5476)
	Direct 561-533-7704
E-mail orders:	orders@HolismPublishing.com or
	www.HolismMovement.com
Postal orders:	Holism Publishing
	PO Box 3385
	Palm Beach, FL 33480-3385
	U.S.A.

Name: _____

Address: _____

City: _____State: _____ Zip: _____

Country: _____

Telephone: _____

E-mail address: _____

❏   YES, I want _____ copies of Holism Movement

❏   Check or money order enclosed

❏   Visa M/C # _____ Exp. Date _____

CVN#_____ Signature _____

Sales tax:	Please add 6.5% for products shipped to
	Florida addresses. ($1.17 per book)

U.S. Shipping: $17.95/book plus shipping: circle choice

❏ Standard (3-7 days): $4.00 first book, $2.00 each additional
❏ Priority/ground (2-3 days): $6.00 first book $3.00 each additional
Other rates (overnight, 2-day, international)
available by phone or website

Please put me on   ❏ mailing list   ❏ e-mail list

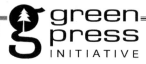

green press
INITIATIVE

Holism Publishing is committed to preserving ancient forests and natural resources. We elected to print this title on 30% postconsumer recycled paper, processed chlorine-free. As a result, for this printing, we have saved:

12 Trees (40' tall and 6-8" diameter)
4,217 Gallons of Wastewater
8 million BTUs of Total Energy
542 Pounds of Solid Waste
1,016 Pounds of Greenhouse Gases

Holism Publishing made this paper choice because our printer, Thomson-Shore, Inc., is a member of Green Press Initiative, a nonprofit program dedicated to supporting authors, publishers, and suppliers in their efforts to reduce their use of fiber obtained from endangered forests.

For more information, visit www.greenpressinitiative.org

Environmental impact estimates were made using the Environmental Defense Paper Calculator. For more information visit: www.edf.org/papercalculator